Healing: An Inner Awakening

Inner Healing Series

Convergences Institute

Healing: An Inner Awakening

David A. Piser CMT, LRT

Writers Club Press
San Jose New York Lincoln Shanghai

Healing: An Inner Awakening

All Rights Reserved © 2000 by David Anthony Piser

No part of this book may be reproduced or transmitted in any form or by any means, graphic, electronic, or mechanical, including photocopying, recording, taping, or by any information storage retrieval system, without the permission in writing from the publisher.

Writers Club Press
an imprint of iUniverse.com, Inc.

For information address:
iUniverse.com, Inc.
620 North 48th Street, Suite 201
Lincoln, NE 68504-3467
www.iuniverse.com

The information, exercises, and procedures contained in this book are based upon the research and the personal and professional experiences of the author. They are not intended as a substitute for consulting with your physician or other health care provider. The publisher and the author are not responsible for any adverse effects or consequences resulting from the use of any of the suggestions, exercies, or procedures discussed in this book. All matters pertaining to your physical and emotional health should be supervised by a health care professional

ISBN: 0-595-14154-4

Printed in the United States of America

Dedication

This first book has taken a great deal of time and patients from many very close to me. Though many have and continue their support, two loved ones come to heart at this moment: Deloris and Dolly. Both taught me how to experience and be in each exquisite moment of life. Thank your for all your love and support; both shall be in my heart always.

EPIGRAPH

Reiki *(Reh-key(JP.) or Ray-key(Eng.))*[1]

A Japanese bio-magneticc modality facilitating physical, emotional, and spiritual healing throughout all life's stages including dying. Reiki is facilitated alone, or during relaxing, integrative, and medical procedures, including surgery.

David A. Piser CMT, LRT
Founder Convergences Institute

[1.] See appendix A

Intentional Healing™

A Western bio-magnetic modality facilitating physical, emotional, and spiritual healing throughout all life's stages including dying. Intentional Healing™ is facilitated alone, or during relaxing, integrative, and medical procedures, including surgery.

David A. Piser CMT, LRT
Founder Convergences Institute

Contents

Dedication v
Epigraph vii
List of Illustrations xi
Foreword xiii
Bibliography xix
Preface xxi
Acknowledgements xxiii
List of Contributors xxv
Introduction xxvii
The Seeds of Health 1
   An Evolution 5
   The Healer's Healing 7
   Truths of Healing 14
   Being Human 18
   How Does it Work? 23
   How Do I Facilitate a Session? 31
   Afterword 55
   About the Author 57
   Appendix A (Reiki: An Interpretation) 59
   Appendix B (Sample intake form) 61
   Appendix C (Healing Protocol) 63
   Appendix D (Our Programs at Convergences Institute) 65

LIST OF ILLUSTRATIONS

Hand Positions (General Session)   35—41
Hand Positions (Self Facilitation)   42—48

All illustrations by Tim B. Muterspaw

Foreword

I initially met David about five years ago, when I decided that I would learn self-defense techniques, something I had intended to learn for the past fifteen years, but kept putting it off. It was a time intuition screams out so loudly, "DO IT NOW!" that ignoring it is out of the question. At the same time, I was searching for a martial arts instructor, I also had decided, for my own personal growth, spiritual growth, and peace of mind; I would begin practicing meditation. (I had been talking to God all my life through prayer, and I felt that it was finally time to learn to be quiet and listen.) With these two things in mind, one of my Anesthesiology partners recommended seeking out Stephen K. Hayes, world-renowned Ninjutsu master, personal bodyguard for His holiness the Dalai Lama, and meditation teacher. Immediately, I scheduled a time to stop by the dojo in hopes that I would be accepted as one of Stephen's students. Excited, I climbed the creaky wooden stairs up a narrow, dimly lit hallway to the dojo. Finally, at the top, and apparently looking rather lost, a tall, slender young gentleman with dark, wavy hair, wire-rimmed glasses, and a thick mustache greeted me warmly. "Hi, I'm David Piser. May I help you?" he asked with a humble and compassionate smile. Instantly, I experienced a peaceful, loving calmness, and I knew that there was something very special about this man.

In addition to having trained extensively in Ninjutsu with Stephen K. Hayes, David had assisted Stephen on many occasions as bodyguard to the Dalai Lama, while His holiness traveled throughout the United States. Initially receiving a higher education degree in Physics,

David had also received training and had gained extensive experience in massage therapy.

It was not until about three months into my Ninjutsu training, that I learned of David's healing abilities, through personal experience. After a particularly rigorous martial arts training session, I noticed a pain in the muscles between my spine and left shoulder blade. Intuitively, David knew that I was experiencing discomfort. Without touching me, he held his hands over the exact area of soreness for a few seconds. I experienced a warm, tingling sensation in the muscle; then gradually the pain subsided. I had not asked him to do that. In fact, I had not even told him I was in pain. He just knew, and without telling me what he was doing, he completely relieved my pain. (I say "he"; but in truth, at the time, I really was not sure WHAT had happened, HOW it happened, or WHO exactly had caused it. However, it was definitely unlike any experience I had ever known.) As a chronic pain management physician, medical doctor, and Anesthesiologist, I instantly recognized the benefit that this "energy" or "what ever it is" could provide for my patients. Turning and asking David what he had just done, he simply smiled compassionately without verbal response. I knew that I had much more to learn.

A few months later, I found that, in addition to the above-mentioned skills, David had become a fifth-degree Reiki master-teacher. Having done some research about bioenergetic healing, and realizing the enhancement that it could bring to western medicine, I invited David to work with me at my pain center and at the hospital. Since that time, David and I have combined our efforts in diagnosing and treating chronic pain and helping to relieve suffering. I must say, his skills in medical intuition, bioenergetic healing, and massage have escalated my practice of medicine to an entirely new level!

During the twentieth century, western medicine has swung its pendulum from one end of the spectrum to the other. Clinicians in the early 1900's, with only rudimentary tools for diagnosing and treating physical illness, focused primarily on the spiritual aspects of healing disease. With improvements in technology and the development of multitudes of medications (particularly during World War I and World War II,) the focus shifted toward using physical modalities (physical therapy, surgery, and medications) to treat physical signs and symptoms of disease. Recognition of the importance of spirituality and the power of the mind decreased, because outcomes using these forms of therapy were much more difficult to measure scientifically. (For example, it is easy to take three groups of hypertensive male subjects ages 45 to 60, give each group a specific dose of Labetalol or placebo, and measure the average decrease in blood pressure with each group. It becomes much more difficult to take the same three groups and measure specific effects of relaxation techniques, visualization exercises, and prayer on blood pressure lowering. How does one actually measure a subject's clarity of visualization or focus during prayer?)

Approximately three decades ago, Norman Cousins, author and editor, developed ankylosing spondylitis, which led to tremendous pain and suffering. Rather than turning to conventional physical therapy and drugs, Norman entertained himself with comedy, and he eventually healed himself through laughter. It was not until the publication of his book, *Anatomy of an Illness,* that clinicians began to once again recognize the importance of the power of the mind in healing the body. Since that time, much support of the mind-body-spirit connection in healing has grown out of works by Bernie Siegel, M.D., M. Scott Peck, M.D., Caroline Myss, Norm Shealy, M.D., Depak Chopra and many others.

Only recently have we begun to scratch the surface in scientifically documenting evidence of the mind-body-spirit connection as a basis for both the development and treatment of disease. As Bernie Siegel, M.D. has stated, "Illness is a reset button" alerting us that we need alter our mental and spiritual paths as well as physically treating our bodies in order to achieve true healing. It has been shown multiple times that stress can trigger or worsen physical disease by inhibiting immune function. According to the Buddhist philosophy, stress, frustration, and suffering are caused by "grasping at self" (fearing loss of something, desiring something that one does not have, or developing depression after loss.) The suffering caused by anger, ignorance, and desire, triggers release of various chemicals in the brain, thus disrupting the normal healthy balance of chemicals in the brain and body. If the suffering is prolonged, permanent physical changes may occur. Meditation and relaxation techniques help decrease the obsession of "grasping at self," thus leading to healing. Certain types of visualization documented by T. D. A. Lingo and Neil Slade have also been shown to help shift focus from self-centered thinking to selfless thinking, escalating the healing processes of the brain/body.

It is known that DNA serves as a blueprint for cellular function and structure, which in turn, determine a person's physical make-up. We are now starting to recognize that this DNA also seems to have an effect on mental function and possibly even spirituality. DNA resonates at a frequency of 52–78 gigahertz when healthy and functioning properly. This creates an electric field different from that created by damaged DNA. DNA repair mechanisms are enhanced in stable individuals with healthy neurochemical balances (discussed above), good nutrition, proper rests and exercise, and avoidance of environmental toxins. Research is now being done with bio-magnetic healers who can alter energy fields around a subject, thus affecting DNA resonance frequencies. Specifically how this works is unknown. Dr. Eric Scott Pearl is the acknowledged instrument through which Reconnective Healing–an evolved form of bio-magnetic healing–is unfolding and being introduced to the world. He once described himself as a form of conduit, a light in prism whose energy blends with that of his patients, goes up to the Universe, and returns to them with an appropriate response. He described it this way: "I am not the healer, only God is the healer, and for some reason, whether I'm a catalyst or a vessel, an amplifier or intensifier, pick your own word, I'm invited into the room." When thanked by one of his patients for healing her, Dr. Pearl responded, "It's like this...It's as if you've just had a wonderful chocolate malted, and you're thanking the straw."

David Piser describes his own work in bio-magnetic healing much the same way as Dr. Pearl. In addition to his success with bio-magnetic healing, David's accuracy as a medical intuitive is outstanding. Over the past four years of working with him in medical practice, David's accuracy of medical diagnostic intuition has surpassed ninety percent.

In discussing the interactions of mind/body/spirit, a well-known medical doctor once described personal health metaphorically as a three-legged stool. If one of the legs is broken, the stool will fall. All three legs must be functioning properly for the stool to serve its purpose. The concept clearly shows that mind, body, and spirit each must function properly for a person to experience optimum health. However, the analogy of individual legs of a stool might mislead one to believe that the three aspects of humanness are separate and that ailments of each aspect can effectively be treated separately. Unfortunately, this is precisely what western medical practitioners have attempted to do over the past three decades. With this system, the patient usually finds himself or herself with one or more health care practitioners managing physical signs and symptoms of disease, other practitioners managing mental aspects of disease, and yet other professionals managing the spiritual aspects. In the vast majority of cases, the patient is left to somehow miraculously integrate and balance the benefits of all three. By virtue of its nature, bio-magnetic healing serves as a mechanism for healing mind, body, and spirit as one "whole" entity, rather than three separate segments of the same entity. For this reason, I believe that bio-magnetic healing shall and will become a standard practice in our medical culture of the twenty-first century.

One final note to you, the reader: Look at yourself as a "whole" entity, rather than as three separate segments—mind, body, and spirit. Take responsibility for your dis-ease, whatever it might be, and use it to stimulate your own personal and spiritual development. Remember that change is what elicits pain and suffering triggered by grasping at self. The pain and suffering necessitate learning, which in turn teaches us to change our internal structure to bring about peace, hence, the paradox of change and pain. Life is a series of lessons through which we learn, mature, and progressively grow closer and closer to achieving inner peace and harmony with the universe, (i.e. total spiritual, intellectual, and physical maturity.) Use this book as a guide, first, for your own personal growth and maturity, and then use your experience to help others. Just as one thought can affect the entire body, so can one enlightened individual make a difference in society.

Glenda Dahlquist, M.D.

July 26, 2000

Bibliography

Lappe', Marc: ***The Tao of Immunology–A Revolutionary New Understanding of Our Body's Defenses.***
Plenum Press, (New York), 1997.

Lingo, T. D. A.: ***The Self-Transcendence Workbook.*** Neil Slade, (Denver), 1998.

Pearl, Eric: http://www.drericscottpearl.com. Word Wide Web site 1999-2000h.

Moyers, Bill: ***Healing and the Mind.*** Doubleday, (New York), 1993.

Myss, Caroline: ***Anatomy of the Spirit.*** Three Rivers Press, (New York), 1996.

Myss, Caroline and Shealy, C. Norman: ***The Creation of Health.*** Forward by Bernie Siegel, M.D., Three Rivers Press, (New York), 1993.

Siegel, Bernie S.: ***How to Live Between Office Visits.*** Harper Collins Publishers, (New York), 1993.

Slade, Neil: ***Frontal Lobes Supercharge.*** Neil Slade, (Denver), 1998

Slade, Neil: ***Cosmic Conversations.*** Neil Slade, (Denver), 2000

Thondup, Tulku. ***The Healing Power of the Mind–Simple Meditations for Health, Well-being, and Enlightenment.*** Shambhala, (Boston), 1996.

Preface

Taking responsibility for one's health has become very popular in the past few years. This is easily seen from the mass of books, videos, and teachers who aggregate in the name of holistic health, or integrative health. This book explores an interesting aspect of integrative health—esoteric healing, or healing from within who you are. A healing, which takes place in the core of who you are as a person. The very nature of esoteric healing, on the surface, contradicts the procedures and protocol of the modern scientific method. Because of the nature of this form of healing this book, in addition, explores a concept of health through a clear awareness, or recognizing your personal perspective or intent of lifestyle.

"Healing: An Inner Awakening", is a work with two very important sections. The first half explores how our quality of life reflects our inner interpretations and habits. It suggests our personal perspective can create a healthier or more balanced experience of life. The second half looks at the mechanics of facilitating a session. What is esoteric healing, How does it work, and How can I facilitate a session are discussed.

"Healing: An Inner Awakening" is a sort of "How to" and "What is it" as far as Intentional Healing™, Reiki, or any form of bio-magnetic healing. The first section is a guideline for facilitators, and good background for anyone interested in personal refinement. If you are medical profession or a mom dealing with a full house of children, the first section introduces some food for the heart and soul.

This book is written so it can be understood without cover to cover reading. Though to understand the complete perspective of this work read it completely, then try some of the exercises. May you enjoy this work and the remainder in the series.

Acknowledgements

I would like to thank Glenda Dahlquist MD for her courageousness. Doctor Dahlquist has opened the allopathic, modern Western medical, world to a controversial and scrutinized modality of esoteric healing, also known as energetic healing, or spiritual healing. This form of integrative medicine is filled with misunderstanding though Doctor Dahlquist embraces it in an attempt in creating a better quality of life for her patience and patience of physicians who consider Intentional Healing™ as an option for their patience's health care plan.

I would also like to thank those students and clients who have assisted in the creation of this first volume. With out those who desire bringing greater brightness to the world and those seeking methods for increasing brightness in their life this book and knowledge would lay dormant and useless. I thank you for all your persistent support.

I would also like to thank Tim B. Muterspaw who provided the illustrations. This is his first time creating illustrations for a non-fiction book, and in an uncanny manner knew exactly what I needed before I began describing anything, thank you and good luck in your life's journey.

Thank you Ann for your trust, patience, and love. My life's work takes me beyond what most would call typical.

LIST OF CONTRIBUTORS

Glenda M. Dahlquist MD…Foreword
Tim B. Muterspaw…illustrations

Introduction

Can humans heal through a sheer thought or intention of healing? Supporting anecdotes and evidence slip by, casually ignored. This book covers a brief, possible description of how one can heal another beginning with a single compassionate thought. This exploration is grounded in simple physical science and 2500 years of Eastern understanding of human experience. Personal awareness and insight are key to health and healing, hence the term esoteric healing. These topics are presented in a non-sectarian manner. They are just a few ideas and exercises for those wishing greater understanding, fun, and something for practitioners to play with.

There are forces that baffle current scientific understanding. Particle behavior remains a hot topic in modern physics. How certain viruses and bacteria elude modern drug therapies, remains baffling. Even the human body's regenerative and immune systems remain in question. The topic covered here is under much skepticism and a topic of current research. This book offers a hypothesis for the mechanics of bio-magnetic healing. However, only continued exploration will yield a scientific explanation of our full healing ability.

As esoteric healers the time has come to work along with Western medical practitioners and one another creating integrity and acceptance. Whatever your method's name, Intentional Healing™, Reiki, bio-magnetic healing, or Healing Touch™, ultimately the goal is the same, balance—healing. Speaking to the mainstream society must be our goal, rather converting the mainstream to our needs. Let us dwell on our similarities and promote a brighter and healthier community for all.

The volumes following this manual will explore topics introduced in greater depth and detail. This manual yields greater understanding and language bridging the span between the every day and intangible. May this volume inspire explorations of self and all that is.

The Seeds of Health

Prevent Anger Today

Attachment and un-clarity creates a very uneasy sense within us. Sometimes these feelings intrude upon our life perspective: right from wrong, good and bad. Most people experience anger as loosing control. Venting anger is great sometimes, but imagine transforming this rage into a positive motivating energy. Remove the seeds and roots of anger from your life now. What is it you want in life? Plant the seeds of happiness within yourself; cultivate what you want in life. Knowing what you want is the first step in avoiding most anger. Then learning to communicate it and do what we must to bring it into reality lessens our sense of frustration. Foresight is a wonderful tool against destructive anger.

Prevent Worry Today

Worry is a trap encouraging a hindering attachment. Worrying is a sort of trick we play on ourselves. I think I am preparing without truly doing so! Knowing my mind is busy; I easily ignore anything I choose. Ask your self, "Can I change this situation?" If so then get to it! If not, the only thing to do is maintain your clarity, awareness, and insight during these uncomfortable moments.

Be Grateful Today

Appreciation of the here and now establishes a connection with that special inner sense of yourself. "Here and now!" rather the "than and was", or the "there and when," here and now is all anyone possess. Grasping and attaching heart and mind to past successes, a lost moment, or living for what may be the greatest day, produces pain and suffering. Greener pastures across from the here and now draws hearts overlooking the beauty and blessings now in our hearts. Being aware of this moment unveils a sense of appreciation and happiness. A sense too often overlooked, or overwhelmed.

Work Hard Today

We take time to care for our physical body and needs every day. We bathe and clothe it. Spend days creating money for greater comforts. At times, we live life as plants, moving from uncomfortable shady areas to bright sunny spots. Take a few moments to center, focus on that inner self, that me inside, and listen. What do I honestly need, and what do I honestly say to myself in my own mind and heart? Work diligently maintaining your inner awareness. Make a commitment to your inner centered self. Fulfill the visions of your heart diligently, not those of someone else.

Be Kind to Others Today

We generate our experience through thoughts, words, and actions. People tend to stay clear if you always complain or speak in the negative. Smiling creates a world of friendship and connection. Is what someone said to you really that important to retaliate? Maybe ask a friend if you appear approachable and friendly with others. I rather experience a world filled of supportive friends. Would you?

An Evolution

Touch is the oldest human method for restoring health and balance. Ancient healing doctrines describe cause and effects of such treatment. However, evidence is found in every life, during almost every experience of compassionate touch, whether physical, emotional, and/or spiritual.

Reiki is a Japanese form of esoteric healing. This system stems from esoteric Buddhist and Taoist teachings. Mikao Usui sensei[2] discovered this system in the 1900's. The founder discovered a healing affect through esoteric mind science methods. His training under Tendai Mikkyo gave access to such esoteric experiences, practice, and information. Though it is mentioned, Usui sensei latter continued his practice of Mikkyo under the Shingon sect. Still to this day, there are diverging stories of Reiki's history, even with recent practitioners uncovering valid proof of its history in Japan.

Usui sensei provided access to many individuals in his lifetime. Latter Hawatha Takata, an attuned teacher, introduced Reiki to the West via Hawaii.

As Western medical physician's interest increases in integrative health techniques, these systems must gain trust amongst the Western medical community and society. Reiki/Intentional Healing™ being a relatively new method in our country must work with the current Western medical establishment, provide a consistent and professional

---

[2] Sensei-A proper title used for a teacher of doctor in Japan.

training sequence, and promote an integrative relationship with Western medical practitioners and the main stream community.

Intentional Healing™ is a system maintaining Usui sensei's integrity, while providing greater access for all born in a Western culture. Preserving the traditions, experiences, and meaning of the Eastern mind science inherit of Reiki. Intentional Healing™ yields this powerful esoteric healing system in a non-religious, though very spiritual, method using common Western language.

Intentional Healing™ finds its roots in Reiki and Eastern mind science. The first goal is awakening or manifesting a grounded reason for perusing esoteric healing, and giving simple and effective tools for the practitioner in facilitating balance for all. Intentional Healing™ is more than a system of techniques and other worldly terminology. It is a system provoking growth, awareness, and balance in its practitioners.

The Healer's Healing

Regardless of certification, license, even knowledge, and experience facilitators operate from a human experience. Being human facilitators are inherently susceptible to all the emotional, spiritual, and physical traps, shortcomings, and ailments of humans. Being an energetic healer requires the greatest of personal responsibility. The utmost attention towards personal balance–health–is very necessary.

All forms of energy or esoteric healing systems work within natural universal Principles, not humanly perceived and limited explanations. Therefore the healer's first priority is listening and taking responsibility for one's personal health, one's personal healing.

A healer's attunement[3] or realization of healing is a lifetime gift. However, attachment, aversion, and ignorance, the human spirit's poisons, affects a facilitator's clarity and intent. These *poisons* affect the spirit as dents alter a satellite dish's reception, or how a scratch or smudge changes a mirror's reflective quality. The healer's cure is personal awareness tempered by the appropriate actions and motivations that create health within the healer's personal experience.

Reiki and Intentional Healing™ work through and heal all it meets. However there are some considerations for a "less effective" session. First, the receiver must be receptive. The receiver and facilitator are partners. If the recipient is just "checking things out" there is a lack of commitment, which is crucial to esoteric healing. It is the equivalent of

---

[3] An attunement is any event that alters a person's perspective in life, an epiphany. (i.e. Birthday, Baptism, Marriage, Completing an exam, even dying.)

getting married just for the experience of being married. Trust, connection, and a commitment to one's own personal healing are very important. Another critical concern is the healer's physical, emotional, mental, and spiritual health. The facilitator's personal health directly effects the session's quality. Heal self, pay attention to self, and be aware of what is happening inside and about. Listening to heart or who some call God, taking care of our bodies through diet and exercise, and leaning more about self and the world produces a personal empowering well being. The facilitator's health, on all levels, greatly effects a sessions quality. Imagine meeting a surgeon who must operate on your body. Imagine this surgeon greeting you smoking a cigarette, grossly unfit, speaking with slurred speech, and unable to make eye contact, does this surgeon gain your confidence and respect? Creating an outwardly apparent well being demonstrates the quality of self and the recommendations offered as esoteric healers.

Beginning Your Journey

This sense of well being requires more than a simple attunement or magic pill. No one can just give it away; it is a very personal and intimate discovery from within self. Maintaining a sense of clarity, insight, and spontaneity requires a lifetime of discrete awareness and action, or idleness. This requires an understanding of self and the operation of the world about and within. Life itself prompts and encourages personal exploration. During this intimate and personal journey, we come upon a very powerful tool—meditation.

What is meditation? Why should you meditate? How should you meditate? Meditation coupled with intellectual pursuit reveals unrealized textures in life. As a child, tools for the intellectual exploration of the world abound, and spiritual exploration is left for Sunday lectures and prayers in dire times. Prayer is taught as a method of communicating with all that is, but personal spiritual exploration is left to intellectual pursuits. Meditation promotes inner growth. This growth prompts greater exploration. Meditation reveals new possibilities of expansion, understanding, and living in the moment. It is a tool assisting with challenging boundaries and inner listening yielding clear understanding and personal refinement.

Meditation is a mental state of being completely aware of the present moment. No attachments or mind chatter, a deeper more connected sense of being overcomes common thought. It is not a zoned or spaced out sensation. Checking today's grocery list, planning tomorrow's attire, or recalling a comedy show is called wandering through thought. Meditation is a clear focused, expanded sense of presence. There are many levels of meditation. The lightest is a greater awareness of your surroundings. The deepest is a synergy of connection and awareness of the moment when the conventional sense of self dissolves. Dissolving into another as a single point; the act of observing, the sense of the state of awareness, and the observed disappear.

Relaxing, focusing, energizing, exploring how the "automatic pilot operates", or altering patterns of accomplishment in life are a few applications for meditation. These are good goals for intent-full meditation, but beginning proves difficult with such a vast choice of styles available. The best position to start is the beginning. How does one maintain intricate visual patterns in mind without the proper concentrative muscle? Do body builders begin lifting two hundred pound weights? New bodybuilders start with a manageable weight working towards their goal. Meditation is the same as acquiring any skill. It requires practice, patience, and determination.

Meditation is a learn-able skill. Some may say it is too difficult to concentrate longer than a moment or physically it may be too demanding. These reasons may be valid, but they are not good enough for dispelling an exercise that enhances your life experience. Would you continue a habit known to kill you or your loved ones? Ask yourself, "What bit of wisdom or desire is attempting to create itself through this habit?" If you understand the benefit or heartfelt reason for any habit, a desire for creating a more positive method for expressing this inner desire can present itself.

Exercising produces stronger muscles and physical endurance. Training is arduous and discouraging at times, but the benefits outweigh the alternative. The same is true with meditation training. As periods of meditation increase, so will concentration and endurance for sitting still. Life becomes more direct and engaging as your skill in this art matures. Unseen options come forth as the rational mind subsides.

It is very important to take time for learning such a valuable life tool. As facilitators, increasing our ability should be our secondary motive for learning meditation. Our primary motivation is creating greater clarity, focus, and confidence. This yields a life filled with compassion, love, fulfillment, and a greater understanding of the truth of "reality."

First, find a comfortable, quiet, and safe place to practice. This could be a favorite chair or in a private garden gazebo. Find an area free from gross distractions. This assists reaching the goal of meditative consciousness. Once your concentrative muscle strengthens, explore using different images, healing aromas, and sound.

The ideal is meditating for a minimum of thirty minutes per session. Just as certain physiological changes begin at the twenty to thirty minute period during physical training the same holds true for the mind. However, beginning with a three hundred second session is best. Imagine your first jogging experience a 25-mile marathon. Phew, this would be discouraging in the least. Shorter sessions build endurance, confidence, and concentrative muscle. They also serve as short vacations during the day.

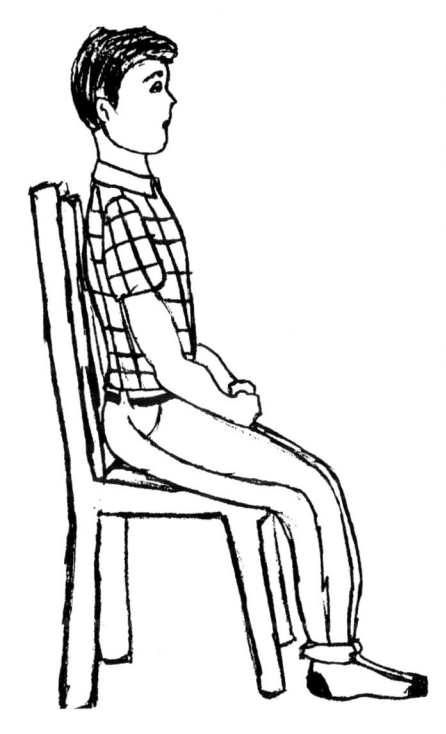

Proper Body Alignment Using a Standard Chair. (Highly recommended)

Be creative in tracking the time of your session. Approximately 21 breaths equal 300 seconds. Find a gentle alarm, not an egg timer; something gentle, a friend, or a set of counting beads. Defining a period yields a sense of accomplishment at the end. It is no more than a reference point. With greater experience, you may lengthen your sessions, or shorten them too.

Sit up; this deters any temptation of taking a nap. Remember your goal is being fully aware—here and now. As athletes warm up their bodies so must meditators. This reduces urges to fidget during your session, and increases the amount of oxygen and nutrients to our body. This promotes a sense of alert awareness while sitting still. Speak with your physician for a general set of stretches if you experience any form of pathology. Otherwise, enjoy a short routine of stretches that open the five major areas of the body. These are: both hip joints, both shoulder joints, and the neck. There is a seated routine, which opens the four major energy centers of the body. (Investigate a stretching routine that suites you best.)[4] The point is increasing blood flow, limbering your muscles, and increase alertness.

---

[4] Consult with your physician before attempting any physical exercise.

Bodies awake and prepared, begin shifting your attention gently inward. Take a few deep breaths filling your abdomen. Breathing in this manner allows the full use of the air or energy surrounding us. This method of breathing completely fills your lungs with air. Enjoy the breath for the next few moments. With eyes open, feel the breath moving in and out of your body. With the next breath, hold it. Allow your chest and shoulder muscles to relax around your inflated lungs. Now, release the breath. This encourages an anatomically straight posture. Adjust your chin so it is parallel with the floor, and your shoulders are over your hips. A properly aligned seat or skeletal structure smoothes each breathe. Your breath should move effortlessly in and out of your body, removing another external distraction.

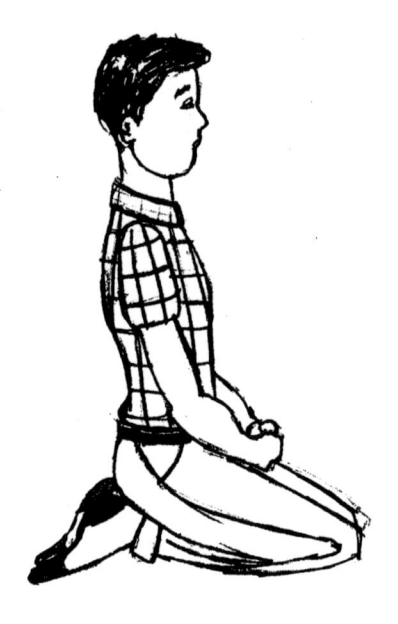

This position is commonly associated with Eastern cultures. It is show with the proper body alignment for meditation and comfort.

Gently close your eyes. Imagine your senses reaching out into the room. Explore the first sense that attracts you. If it is your hearing, explore every sound you hear. Explore each and any aromas, taste any flavors, experience, and reach out with your senses. Gently exploring all your sense, which are usually taken for granted. Explore the room with your senses as a child investigates a fresh spring meadow.

Continuing, turn your conscious mental awareness inwards. Place your attention on the breath; gently turn your focus inward. With each inhalation and exhalation fix all your attention, awareness, and focus on your experience of the breath. This allows your breath to serve as a bridge into meditative awareness.

Your mind or body may beckon you back during the exercise. When it does, quietly say in your heart, "Not now, Here now..." Allow your attention to drift back to your breath. If a sever pain is experienced or a great urge to move arises, do so and return to your breath. Coordinating the words, "Here," with each inhalation and, "Now," upon exhalation may provide a gentle reminder of your goal for present in the "moment-ness".

Reverse this process to return to a conscious state. Place your full attention on the breath then explore the room with your senses. Once you have expanded your senses stretch your shoulders and body, feel the floor. Remind yourself you are back in the room. Lower your head so your eyes open to the floor. How do you feel now? How did you feel before this exercise? Maybe you have a new insight, new energy, or are ready for a nap. Whatever your experience calls for, you will feel at this moment.

This simple exercise allows you to plunge the depths or breach the heights of subconscious awareness. Practicing this exercise yields greater mental concentration, physical revitalization, and preparation for advanced meditative work, and a "centered-ness" you can carry throughout your life.

Truths of Healing

How can I refine my experience of life? "Well I'm ok, it's everyone else who disrupt the natural beauty of *MY* life!" an old friend continually murmurs under his breath, with each breath. For my friend's sake, let us look at the inner aspects of healing. Earlier the ideas of the poisons of spirit were introduced as the cause of illness. (i.e. attachment, aversion, and ignorance.) Also introduced are the conditions that ripen these causes: lifestyle, diet, seasons/period of life, and unseen factors (genetic, viral, mind etc…). With the practice of meditation and exploring these ideas of healing some roots for disease can be plucked from our fertile soil of mind, rather heart.

Perspective

Life's experience is filtered by relative or personal perspective. Our individual tastes create a sense of pleasure or dis-ease. Our perceptions affect our well being, our balance. This is not to say personal preference or desire is necessarily wrong. If we are aware this personal taste creates difficulty for self and others and accept the responsibility and consequence of this preference, fine. Otherwise being unaware creates a sense of unhappiness from "unknown" sources. This seed grows making the recognition of happiness in life more difficult. Yes, in life there are naturally occurring unavoidable events: death, illness, aging, even birth. Though accepting and acknowledging them, doing what we can to reconcile with these natural events, without disguising them, prevents distractions from the more important issue of the moment. Take a moment and recall a small event in life that causes displeasure, maybe a dog barking, or an aggressive co-worker? Whatever that small displeasure, look at it from a fly's perspective from a corner of the room. Do this from a meditative state. What you call agitating may become rather humorous from the fly's perspective.

Aversion & Attraction

Desires, wants, and needs create opportunities for growth. Growth produces change, and change promotes growth. Some desire may require ridding our life of something we have, and it usually includes getting something that appears far from our life. Adding new things in our life and "cleaning out" our lives sometimes is the root of our pain. We want a happy and pleasurable life, and in today's disposable society, we think getting the newer model is the answer for our ills. A new car or a new romantic relationship just may bring the happiness we seek.

Take a moment, again from a meditative state, and look at what you want or wish to throw out. Ask yourself four simple questions:
1) "How will keeping this in my life create a sense of happiness?"
2) "Will getting rid of it create a sense of happiness?"
3) "Do I already have what I say I need in life?"
4) "Is what I need to get rid of truly existent in my life?"

Cause and Effect

If your diet were primarily donuts, coffee, soda, and ice cream, would you always feel awake aware and alert? Would you feel tuned into what is going about you? Maybe for the term of the glucose rush, but the long term result of such a diet is disaster. What you honestly put into something you more than likely know what to expect later in time. Imagine answering every question anyone asks in the negative. "Hay you look great today!" "Yea, ah what do you want?" Do you think this would attract happy motivated people into your life?

However, sometimes it appears you did not get what you should have from your efforts, or did you? Quietly review the situation. Is your heart's intention supported by what you ask or say? Do your actions and work support or create your inspired goal? Ask yourself, "Do you generate the results you want from life?" If not its time for at least one small change in what you are doing. Getting out of bed five minutes earlier could be your golden key.

Healthy Habits

These eight habits create an overall healthier experience of life. On one level, they promote a greater sense of ethics, concentration, and wisdom. These habits create a natural awareness of life and self, promoting a healthier experience of life on all levels.

1) Clear Understanding
2) Clear Thought
3) Appropriate Speech
4) Appropriate Action
5) Appropriate Livelihood
6) Honest Effort
7) Honest Mindfulness
8) Honest Meditation/Concentration

Healing Tools

Sanmitsu is an Eastern concept unlocking the fullest experience of our life. Sanmitsu translates as triple or three secrets. The honest practice of the three secrets creates clarity, happiness, and well being. The tools for this practice are: proper thought or intention, proper speech or word, and proper actions or deed. Our true thoughts or intent must be clearly known, especially as facilitators. Our speech must reflect the intended goals or thoughts, and each action supports our intention and speech. In other words, our heart's intent should reflect in our mental thoughts, our speech, and our actions.

> Close your eyes, relax your shoulders. Rest your hands gently on your thighs or lap. Take a few deep full breathes. Gently recall all the people you share your life with. As faces come and go, release them. Now recall what material items you have in life. Again, make note then release. Look at what you do in life, career, and daily activities. Allow each impression to move through your mind unhindered without any judgment. Take a deep breath, now ask yourself a simple question, "Am I happy with my life?" Gently reflect on your answer.

Thought, speech, and action, each must correlate with our intended goal. It all sounds so easy so why is it is so difficult in practice? Every day, take inventory. Is my life as I intended it to be today? The present is an ultimate test for past thoughts, words, and actions. As facilitators, as human beings this practice becomes of greatest importance in facilitating and living life. If your life is not what you want, then whose life are you living?

Being Human

Within our system the essence of human-ness unfolds in a five fold dynamic of synergistic compliments. All our habits for success and shortcomings are revealed in a trail guide of the human spirit. A guide of a dynamic tapestry spun with each breath. Understanding it unleashes the fullness of human experience.

The Roku Dai[5] stems from an eastern mind science Usui sensei is connected with. It differs from the more widely known Go-Gyo. The Go-Gyo or the Taoist Wu-hsing deals with relationships, the seasons of life, and the process of cycles, their creation, or inhibiting. The Roku-Dai exposes our natural human tendencies. The Roku-Dai assists with recognizing areas of true strength and great potential. Viewing our self with deeper clarity supercharges our experience of life.

The first quality deals with a sense of knowing, both intellectual and spiritual. This knowing encourages a meaningful connection with self and the perceived outer world. The next quality deals with a sense of vision, abundance, and empowerment. This vision inspires accomplishment. Next is a desire for an authentic connection, compassion, passion, and love. Connection and passion encourages an authentic understanding of self and the world. Accomplishment or the sense of personal importance in life is vital. This part sees the vision and relents

---

[5] Roku Dai translates as the great or high 6. The sixth element is mind. Since the mind experiences these other qualities, it is "seen" as an invisible quality to our model.

tills its manifestation. The final is the sense of wholeness, a sense of fulfillment and completeness.

In short, let us call these qualities: Inner Knowledge, Vision, Compassion, Accomplishment, and Fulfillment.

Inner Knowledge:

This is the desire for recognizing truth. Each person desires their belief or understanding of self and the world is true. How does an authentic understanding and acceptance of your life compare to living an elaborate dream?

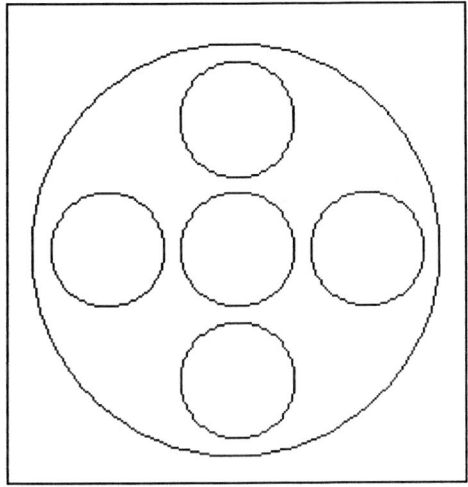

The Roku Dai's schematic begins with Inner knowledge at the bottom most quadrant, moving in a clockwise direction, then moving into the center from the Accomplishment quadrant.

Vision:

The quality of desire for value, abundance, direction, and integrity in life creates a sense of vision. This is the reason why the path is traveled. It is a desire for a quality of life based on dreams and hopes held dear to our heart. Would you enjoy a life moving, living towards an envisioned goal, or a life full of aimless wandering, devoid of structure or guidance aimed at personal fulfillment?

Connection:

The artist within beholds the need and appreciation for direct experience, love, and creativeness, a need for being in touch. Experiencing compassion, being compassionate, and being passionate about life creates the desire of being in touch with self and the world. How would a life of solitary confinement prove against a life rich with loving friends and family?

Accomplishment:

A quality or wish for inclusion in life. A driving force causing the discovery of a personal role in life above daily chores, and enacting more methods of accomplishment. Imagine a life of purpose and ability versus emptiness and difficulties. Which seems more appealing?

Fulfillment:

Each person's desire for peace in life creates the urge for balance or fulfillment. This urge motivates each person towards greater personal realization and actualization. Regrets and dormant dreams create lack though at times inspire us in unveiling the clear light experience of heart, of mind, of life. Which would you desire: a life of despair and vacancy or a life lived in confidence and peace.

Exploring your World

This exploration requires asking yourself a few questions from a relaxed and centered state of mind.
1) What do I want in life?
2) Am I fulfilling my vision, and does it bring value to others?
3) Am I in touch with others, and communicate what I need?
4) Am I skillful acquiring what I need, and do I assist others?

5) **Am I happy with my life experience overall?**

Choose one question per week devoting a few moments every day. Begin this exercise with a shortened breathing exercise from the previous chapter.

> Close your eyes placing your hands, palms open and facing down, on top of your thighs. Listen closely to any sound in the room. After a few deep breaths, slowly shift your sense of awareness and attention to your breathing. How does it feel to breathe? Does the actual movement of your body, or the air moving across your sinuses call your attention? After a few moments, repeat one of the above question quietly to yourself.

Smile and have fun with the exercise. After the exercise, take note of your discoveries, insights, and feelings. Discuss your experience with a friend. Some exercises may appear easier then others; give each question a chance.

Homework for the Spirit

Choose one exercise and make it your theme for that day. Start simple, one day at a time. It is amazing how your wildest dreams come true just attending to the smallest of details in your day.

1) **Learn one new thing today.**
   Broadening our understanding creates tolerance and awareness.

2) **Organize one thing today.**
   Cleaning your desk, closet, or planning a special dinner is a great start. This prepares us for obtaining our goals in life.

3) **Take time to care for yourself, and give someone a smile.**
   Being in touch with others and self allows more easeful communications and greater compassion.

4) **Complete that task you put off a month ago.**
   The accomplishment of the smallest task may be the key to your role in life.

5) **Ask yourself, "Overall am I satisfied right now?" If you are not satisfied, "What one small thing do I need to change?"**
   Satisfaction sometimes is just the realization of what you already have, or enjoying the process of obtaining your goals.

Remind yourself at the beginning of each day of your "assignment." and end each day with an internal review.

—Did I do my assignment for the day?

—How did today turn out?

—If you could change a moment of your day, how would it look?

Be gentle with yourself. Allow each day be an experience of the unfolding of your greatness and brilliance in life.

How Does it Work?

What is difficult to perceive through common physical senses usually evokes mistrust or fear. Intentional Healing™, Reiki, or any form of bio-magnetic healing results from explainable natural occurrences of physical energy. My intention is providing insight and understanding, rather then creating doubts or division. Let us openly explore this quality of human-ness.

What is a bio-magnetic or bio-energetic healing modality?

Bio-magnetic healing modalities promote healing and health through the balancing or realignment of subtle energetic fields. Reiki, Intentional Healing™, and Healing Touch®, for examples, are very powerful yet subtle forms of vibrational or bio-magnetic healing.

Western allopathic physicians employ chemical and surgical influences producing a homeostatic condition within a system. Reiki balances subtle energy fields encouraging inner changes. Healing occurs on a subtle level affecting the more dense physical representation of self, the body.

What is a subtle human bio-magnetic field?

These fields are low level magnetic fields generated through neural stimuli, action potentials. In a standard wire, a flow of electrons creates an electrical field. This varying electric field produces a changing magnetic field. The same principle applies for neurons.

A bee sting or thoughts are examples of a neural or nerve stimulus. Keeping things simple let us look at a bee sting. The bee's sting creates an action potential, or stimulates a nerve(s). The stimulation creates a current of electrons that move along the nerve. More accurately, neural impulses create an electron wave. The electrons generate an electrical and magnetic field surrounding the neuron. This magnetic field then travels away from the nerve and out from the body. This is similar to what happens in wires and radio transmission antennas.

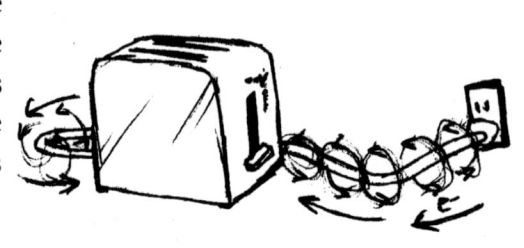

The electromagnetic fields created by and moving from a standard wire is similar to bioelectromagnetic waves propagating from a neuron.

Are these fields detectable?

Modern medical practice use bio-magnetic field detection every day. Electrocardiograms (EKG) and electroencephalograms (EEG) are good examples. The EKG monitors neural impulses, and the EEG monitors gross brain activity. Using sensitive receptors on the skin, these devices detect and report the presence and character of nerve impulses by way of the bio-magnetic field generated by nerves deep inside the body.

Humans perceive these fields, though they exist on the fringe of human sense perception. However, some animals and insects consider these ranges normal. Our brain attempts rationalizing this fringe information the best it can. Sensory capacity, emotional, and physical experiences influence our interpretations. Metaphysical labels embellish these interpretations: auras, charkas, and etcetera. Sensory perceptions, mental, emotional, and spiritual awareness become magical qualities. Though are just normal human qualities. Our range of perception alters the experience of life. Someone with full sense perceptions, brain, or mental abilities compared with an individual without sight, hearing, or with a different approach to reasoning each experience a different texture of life. Environmental experiences vary with sensory perceptions and awareness. Someone may describe a bright and clear day as wonderful, while another person describes it as unpleasant. The other person may suffer from allergies or is photosensitive. For the person experiencing photosensitivity a bright sunny day could be their least favorite day. Our sense perceptions offer different insights and relative truths.

Let us try something fun:

> Close your eyes placing your hands with your palms open and facing down on your thighs. Listen closely to any sound in the room. After a few deep breaths, slowly shift your sense of awareness and attention to your breathing. How does it feel to breathe? Does the actual movement of you body, or the air moving across your sinuses calls your attention? Focus your attention on the feeling in your palms. Are your palms relaxed, tense, sweaty, or dry? Place your total awareness in your palms. Gently, without opening your eyes or too much movement place your hands together, palm-to-palm. How do the palms of your hands feel? Completely focus on the feeling of your palms. After a few moments slowly move your palms slightly apart. Move them about a half-inch apart. What is your experience of the feeling in your palms? After a few moments experiment, move your palms slowly apart and back together. Maintaining a quiet focused intent experience the feeling in your palms.

Allow your hands to rest on your lap. Take a deep breath and shift your focus of awareness from your palms to any sound in the room. Gently allow your eyes to open returning to the place you are sitting.

What was your experience? Did you feel anything, or were you waiting for something to happen? Were you truly doing this exercise? Without loading your experience, know it is valid. Each person is different. The brain attempts interpreting these "odd" signals so interpretations vary. Your experience is your own. Play with this exercise after a heart pumping conversation, a good work out, or just relaxing in peace.

How do subtle Bio-magnetic fields promote healing?

Modern sciences have tools enabling us to see the processes of the brain. These scans reveal words, emotions (intentions), and pathological conditions fire different arrays of neurons. The regions and intensity of neural activity change with intentions and feelings. The bio-magnetic field pattern changes with each stimulation. Remember a though or intention are stimulations.

A drum provides a good example of this phenomenon. A drum produces a sound wave field. The stick hitting the drum is the stimulus creating a series of sound waves, such as how a bee sting or a thought affects a neuron. Many factors affect a drum's tone. The material of the drum's head, the type of mallet, location of and frequency of

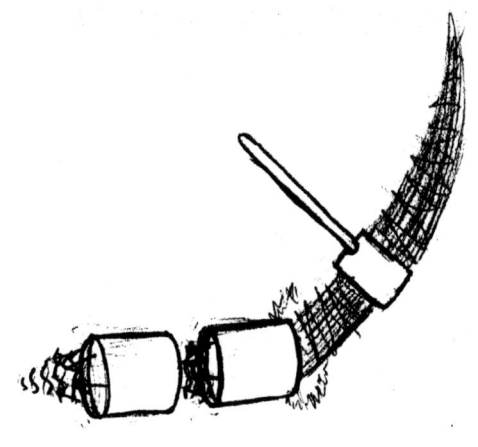

A sound wave is a perfect example of how bio-energetic fields promote balance or healing in others.

strikes, temperature, and size causes different tones. Changing one factor causes a different tone. It is the same for humans, but on a bio-magnetic level.

Lets add another drum to our example. Align their striking surfaces, so they are facing one another. Playing one drum, the untouched drum resonates along with the other. The sound waves or sound field generated from each strike travel through the air, the sound wave's medium. The sound bounces off the *un-played* drum, creating a vibration according to the played drum. Humans affect each other similarly. We affect each other emotionally, physically, and bio-magnetically every day in the same manner. Though in a healing capacity the human bio-magnet/bio-energetic field encourages, and *attracts*, health and balance in our surroundings.

Have you ever heard the old saying, "laughter is contagious" so is sadness, "That guy is a downer". Obviously, our actions and words create our experience of life, which are based upon our thoughts, our intentions, our motivation towards life and ourselves.

Have you ever seen someone who is just so happy and hear others say, "She is just beaming"? Have you ever just wanted to be near someone because, "I don't know, she seems to brighten the room" Our thoughts, coupled with word, and supported with action yield our experience. "She is just beaming!" "He is walking on air!" "She has a contagious smile." are age-old bits describing the influence of intentional or emotional fields. If our thoughts and intentions remain on healing or assisting another this emotional or intentional field affects another as sound waves of a drum effects another drum, and our human eardrums.

A Leap of Faith?

Some systems of bio-magnetic healing, including Reiki, speak of an external healing source of energy. This external source moves through the practitioner into an individual yielding balance—healing. For some this may sound crazy. For others it is a spiritual reality of faith. In other words, others accept in faith that God or who ever you call your Supreme Healer works through some as "healers." If you are not a religious or very spiritual person, it may be a good idea to read on. Otherwise, please do not be offended. The following is a simple explanation based on rudimental science for this idea of healing.

Every thing in life seeks balance. Humans (emotionally and physiologically), weather systems, electric charges–the whole universe seeks balance. Larger negative electrical charges attract smaller negative charges. Water systems seek balance too. Do you remember this simple experiment from elementary school science lab?

> Take a container with a valve and hose attached to the bottom of the container. Place it atop a desk, and fill it to the top with water, oh, the valve is closed. Now take a second container, similar to the first, and place it along the first container but on the floor. Add about a third of the containers volume of water to the second container, and then place the hose of the first buck in it. What happens when you open the valve in the hose between the buckets? The water flows down to the lower bucket until the water levels in each container are of equal volume in both containers. Now connect two hoses to the first container, one tube much wider in diameter then the other. Opening the valves in each tube what happens? The water flows mostly through the wider tube. Why? Because the wider tube presents the path of least resistance, or in human terms is the most skillful method of accomplishing it's natural tendency.

There are many other similar examples as this one. This examples is just a small reminder that all in life seeks balance, and as in the two tube example, in the most efficient and direct method.

A human with an illness is a system seeking balance. Whether the disturbance is a fractured bone, or an invading ragweed particle these circumstances have induced an imbalance in the body's preferred environment. The human body is in a constant flux, as the whole universe, of restoring and maintaining balance.

Everything possesses an electrical charge. Modern sciences indicates what we call matter is mostly space with some energy or forces binding a few pieces of "stuff" creating "solid" objects. Some call this energy chi, ki, prana, or even the breath of God. Some say this is God, ever present. Scientifically the world is a huge energetic field constantly seeking balance. The forms of these energies constantly change, but the amount is constant and dynamic.

Referring back to our bucket example, remember the hose? The facilitator acts as the hose. Setting an intention for healing creates a specific bio-magnetic field around the facilitator creating a conduit of sorts of least resistance for any specific energy for healing. The facilitator's training, attunement, and well being creates an effortless path for this healing energy, or energy which is needed for balance.

What is this healing energy?
Does this healing energy truly exist?

This is a question only you can answer for your self. My personal experience suggests something happens. The exact understanding of the mechanisms of bio-magnetic healing may escape us now. However, balance does occur. This explanation may fall short of the truth or agitate you, or is just too much to digest. You might laugh, snicker, jeer, and even become angry, great! The only recommendation is continue, try a session. Experience tempered with knowledge produces greater understanding–wisdom.

> Find a comfortable chair allowing easy access to a seated friend's head, neck, and shoulders from behind them.

Ask a friend to join you for a fun and balancing experiment. Discuss the concept of bio-magnetic healing with your friend. Ask if they would like to try a session. Once they accept, have your friend sit in the chair. Make sure they are comfortable. Stretch and ask your friend to take a full breath in and release, do the same with him or her. Take a few more deep full breaths together and release. Quietly, set your intention to assist your friend. Gently allow one word repeat in you mind, "HEALING." Gently place your hands, lightly at first, and then allow them to rest on your friend's shoulders just below the base of their neck. Deep breathe in, reciting quietly the word "HEALING." Spend a few moments in this position. Ask your friend to focus on their breathing, while you focus on the word "HEALING." After a few moments pass, gently move your hands from your friend's shoulders. Focus on your breath. Quietly say "RELEASE" in your mind and "THANK YOU" aloud. After a few breathes switch roles with your friend.

Once you have completed this simple session, share your experiences with one another. What did you and your friend experience? If your friends are too busy, try this on your pet or plants. Just allow yourself the time and space for exploration. Maybe you experience is profound, maybe nothing. What ever your experience, it is great! You explored a new concept; you tried something different that is all that matters.

How Do I Facilitate a Session?

Intentional Healing's™ and Reiki's simplicity allows its use at anytime anywhere. Perfect settings for sessions are quiet rooms, crowded malls, busy office areas, and surgical rooms. The simple intention of healing or Reiki begins facilitation.

Each attunement instills a subconscious trigger focusing your thoughts, words, and actions towards healing. The individual becomes a sort of conduit for healing. This requires the need for centering or calming before any session. Take a few full breaths. This focuses and calms the mind creating a greater experience for all involved.

Permission

An individual's permission is needed before a session. In the event someone denies consent acknowledge his or her wishes. Thank them and just be with them. That is if they chose that you be with them. With an individual's agreement, facilitate.[6]

A client intake form is appropriate. In appendix B, a sample intake form is provided. This form offers the practitioner necessary information, and yields consent for facilitation.

During an emergency, the recipient may be unconscious. Immediately call for emergency medical assistance. If you are a trained medical practitioner and trained in Intentional Healing™ or Reiki, facilitate while performing emergency medical procedures. Remember

---

[6] Remember permission is very important legally and morally. To force your will or control over another can result in a return you may wish not deal with.

get help first. The goal is providing the greatest quality of care. Western medicine and integrative medicine each have their place during an individual's healing process. The convergence of these systems creates a more powerful team promoting the healthiest experience in each life.

Then how can someone facilitate while walking through a crowded room, or with someone under sedation, or is unconscious? How is permission granted with no prior contact? Just facilitate with the best of intentions for all involved. Just as someone receiving a smile makes a conscious decision of first noticing then retuning the smile, the same applies here. Each of us has the choice of accepting or leaving something presented, on any level of awareness.

Creating a Healing/Comfortable Space

The session room's environment should promote relaxation and trust. Ideally, the area should be free from as many distractions as possible. The space is best simple and relaxing for anyone who enters. Too many sense distractions can make another feel uneasy. A busy, cluttered, or other worldly environment may "turn off" people requesting a session. Subdue lighting, quiet music, and a comfortable setting is key. Creating a relaxed and safe environment yields a greater trust and openness promoting a wonderful experience.

Surgical rooms, physician's clinics, and emergencies usually do not fit this model. Most patients arriving are already anxious. However, through intent these areas work fine. The environment can be subdued. However, this requires an explanation beyond the scope of this book.

Client Positioning

Ideally, a solid, safe, commercially available massage or energy workers table is best. This allows the client to fully relax into the session. Disrobing is not necessary for any reason, other than you are a professional massage practitioner facilitating bio-magnetic healing during a massage session or medical professionals providing a medical service.

A solid chair is fine if the client is comfortable. This is a good option for anyone feeling uncomfortable lying down or may have physical challenges. A good professionally available massage chair is great. Professional massage chairs work great for on-site sessions, corporate and public demonstrations. Otherwise, a solid, dependable, and comfortable chair works well.

It is important to mention wheel chairs, medical beds, or were ever the person may be is fine. The facilitator always provides for those, whoever and wherever, facilitation is requested.

Ethics

Integrity, professionalism, sincerity, and confidentiality create TRUST! Unless properly licensed or legal in your state, never provide counseling of any kind. Listen and be with this person. It appears from recent discoveries Usui-sensei required his students learn how to be present with the individual. He appears to dissuade counseling, just being with someone.

Never discuss your clients during casual conversation. Respect your clients' privacy. Do not share any confidential information about your clients with friend(s). Not even a client's friends, your client may wish their participation in such sessions be unknown. Respect his or her confidentiality.

Be aware of your intent. A client will sense if your mind is unfocused or misplaced. Have you ever shared time with someone in a rush to leave, but did not verbalize it? Was it very comfortable? If your motives are other then healing, say groceries, money, ego, or a movie the client will notice. The quality of the session depends on your clarity of intent, your clarity of mind.

Be aware of your touch. It does not matter whether you are the same gender or not. This is referring beyond the obvious sexually charged areas. Respect each person's individual personal space.

Our speech is very important. Speak directly and politely. Be honest, considerate, and caring. Off color jokes or brash tones may confuse or scare someone.

Dress comfortable presenting yourself in a professional manner. How can you introduce healing to the world if your physical appearance causes doubt? Be clean, neat, and professional. As esoteric healers, we are here to assist.

Just as thoughts, words, and actions influence esoteric healing on its subtle levels, it affects our obvious physical world. Most individuals create initial opinions and decisions of trust on language and physical appearances. Cultivating the highest expression of language and presence opens trust in new ideas and concepts.

Check out local laws for any requirements for offering bio-magnetic healing. If counseling services are included, or medical treatments, assure your licensing or accreditations are adequate for the state you practice within. It may be a good idea to work with a school that provides some connection with a professional association. Remember, anything that displays integrity, professionalism, and credibility to clients, prospective clients, and our community is great! Whatever creates openness for healing and balance, do it!

The Session

Center your self before and during a session. Practice a short version of the centering meditation from the earlier chapter. Approximately five to ten breaths should be fine. Once centered, allow your mind to rest on the matter at hand—healing. Place all your attention on the person requesting the session. The following pages demonstrate a pattern of hand placements. Remember this is a form. Deviation is fine, as long as you and the receiver are comfortable, and complete at least one expression of the form. These placements correspond with specific meridians and energetic anatomy. Reiki is a head down system. This is fine but trust your intuition[7]. What does this individual need now, at this moment to promote healing, peace, and integrity?

Hand Positions (General Session)

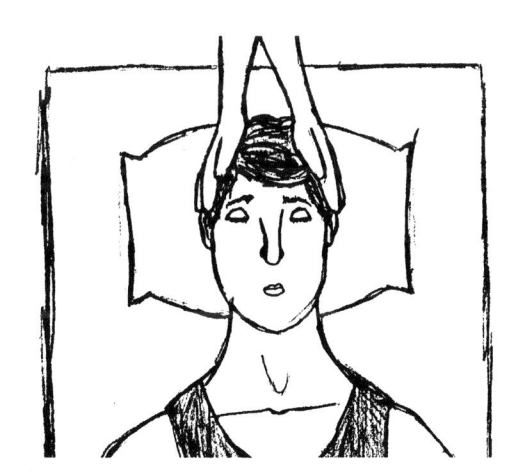

Gently place your hands on your friend as shown. Physical touch is 7th on the healing protocol list, scanning is usually executed before sessions.

Maintain a light and compassionate touch

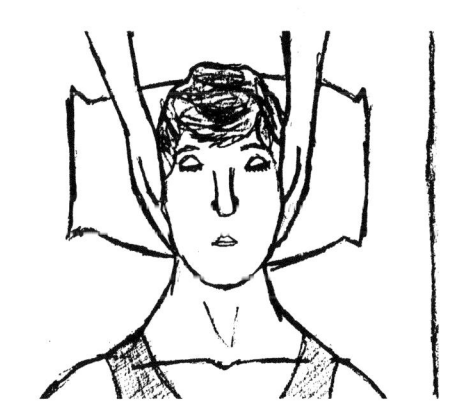

---

[7] Appendix C offers a protocol for each session.

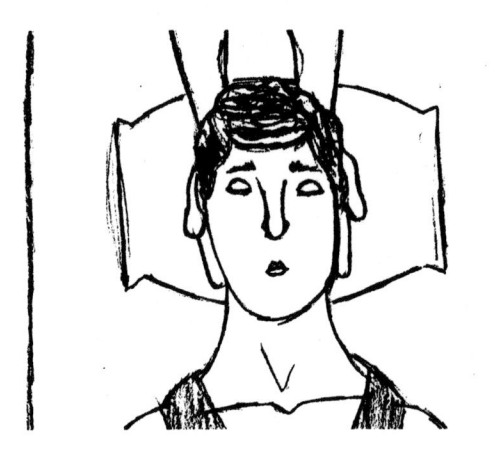

Gently ease one hand at a time under your friend's head. Begin with your fingertips, slipping each hand under the head, cradling their head as shown. Your fingertips should rest at the occipital region of the cranium.

A towel can be placed over your friend's eyes. However, contact is not made with the eyes or eyelids. Your hands should lightly cup over your friends eyes. Though if your client relaxes more with a small hand towel over the eyes that is just fine.

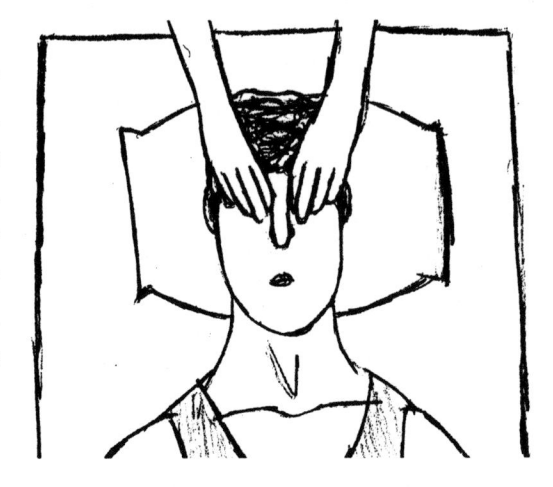

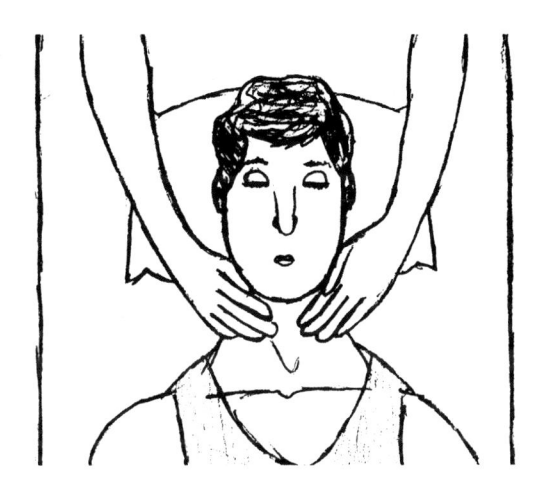

Lightly rest your hands on both sides of your friend's neck. Any pressure can create an uncomfortable feeling or choke your friend.

Remember a relaxed resting hand is key.

Women may feel uncomfortable with this position. If your friend is uncomfortable, place your hands along the top of their shoulders.

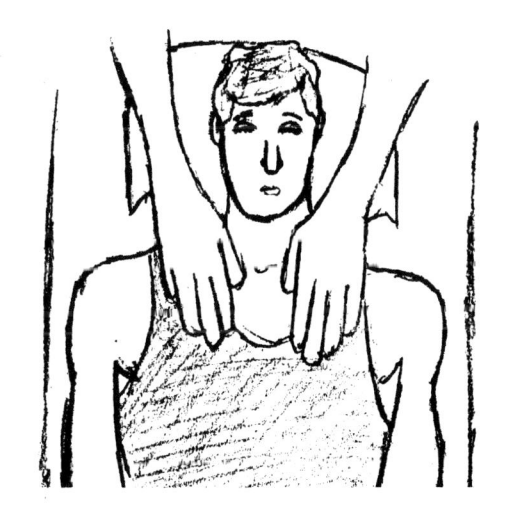

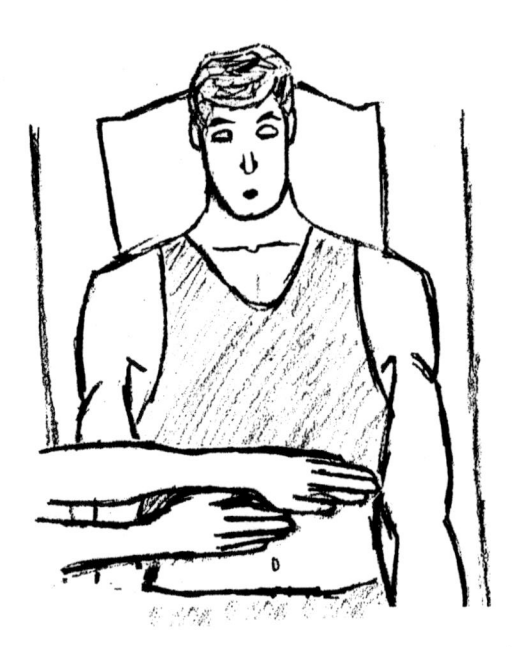

Gently rest your hands along the floating ribs. If your friend is uncomfortable with this touch, allow your hands to rest about one inch above this same area, and remember to focus on your breath.

Being mindful of your friend's comfort, allow your hands to ease on the iliac crest. (The top outer edges of the pelvic bone.)

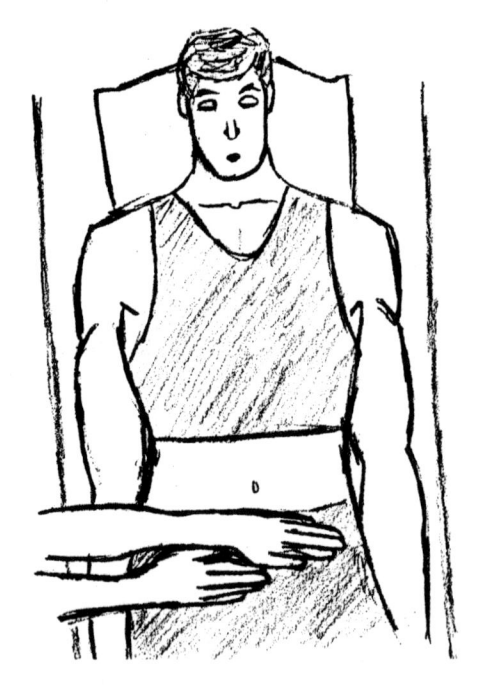

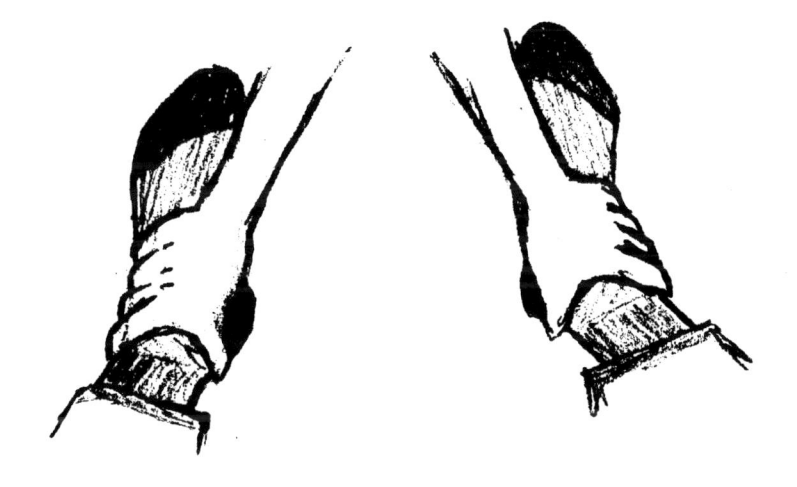

Allow your hands to rest on each knee, one side at a time. Then move and touch your friend's feet as illustrated, then hold each foot one at a time.

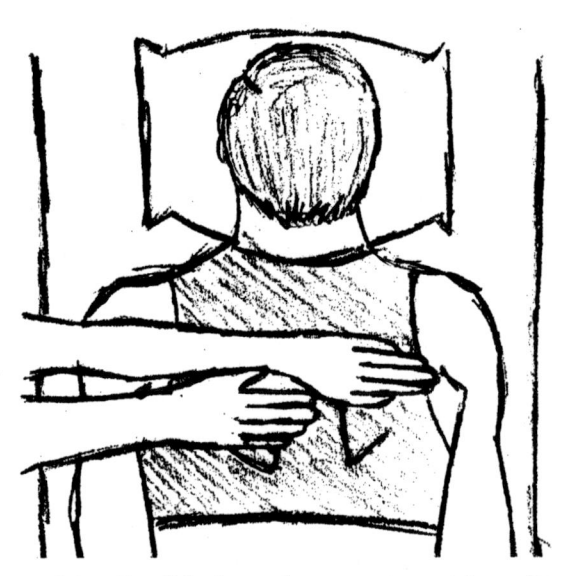

Assist your friend safely into the prone position. (Face down) Begin with both hands resting between the scapulas, the shoulder blades, of your friend then along the bottom ribs of your friend's rib cage.

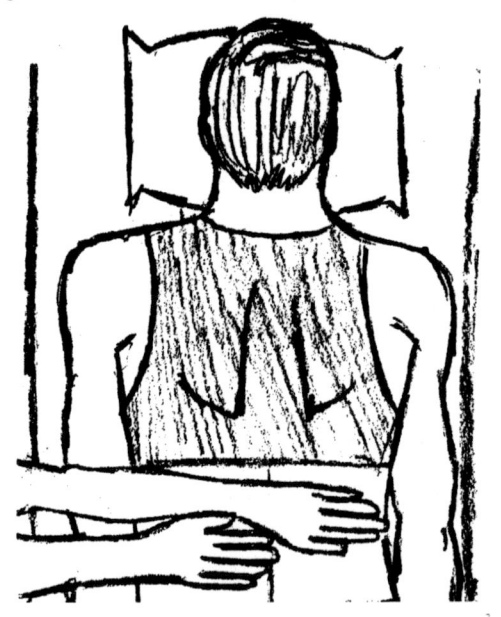

Your hands slowly move to the lilac crest, again monitoring your client's comfort.

With your right hand remaining on the lower back. Allow your other hand to move to the top of your friend's head.

The final position is with both hands over your friend's heart.

Hand Positions (Self Session)

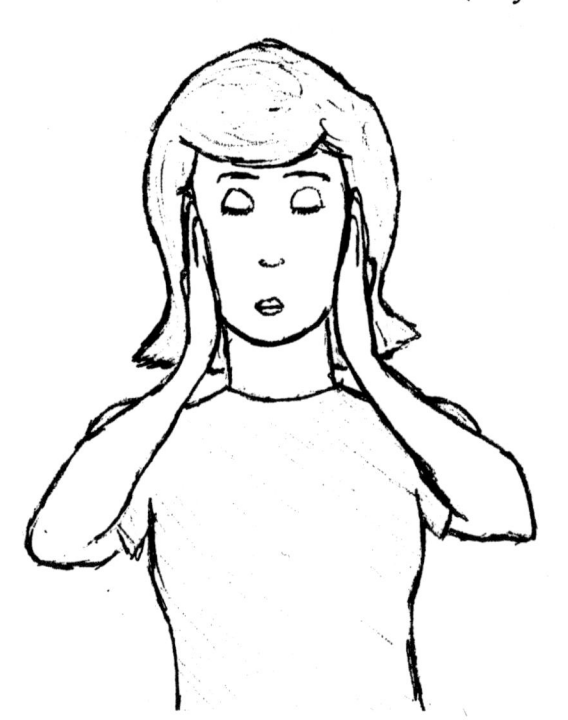

The procedure for a personal session is the same. Maintain a light touch, lift your hands from any areas of pain or discomfort, and maintain your focus on your breathing.

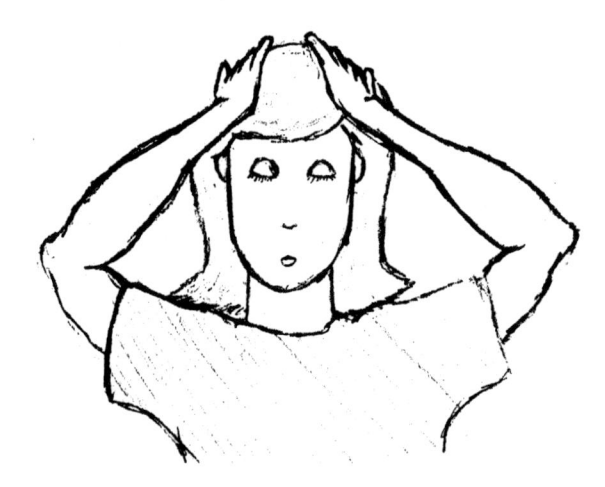

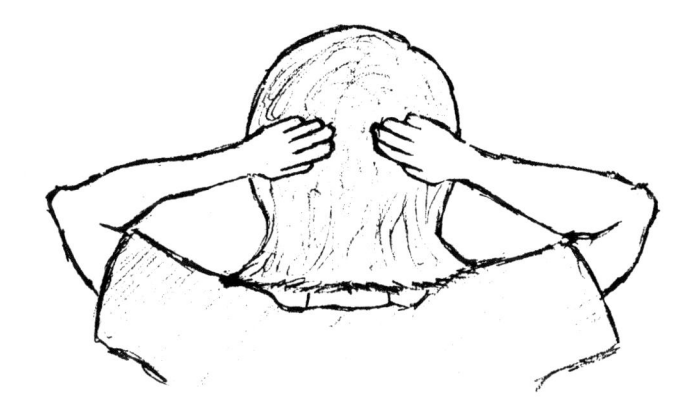

Watch your breath moving in and out from your body.

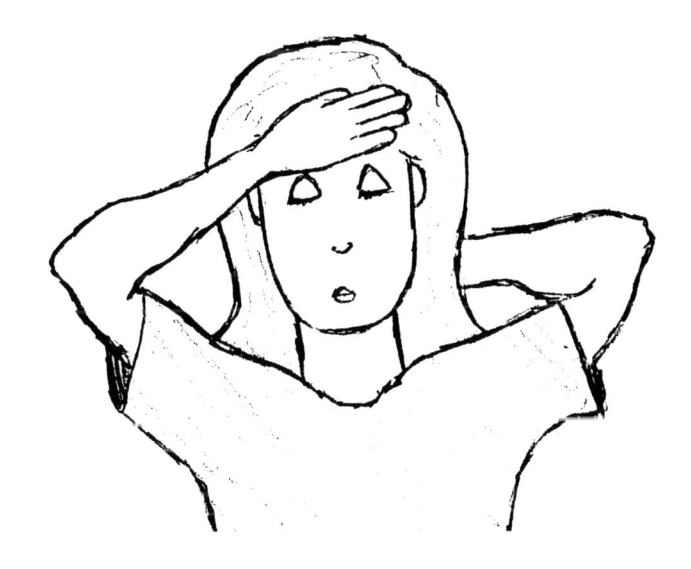

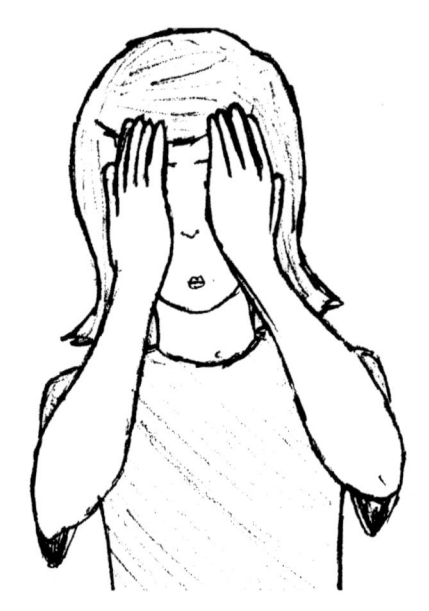

Notice any change in your body? What is the quality of your breath, fast or slow, tense or relaxed?

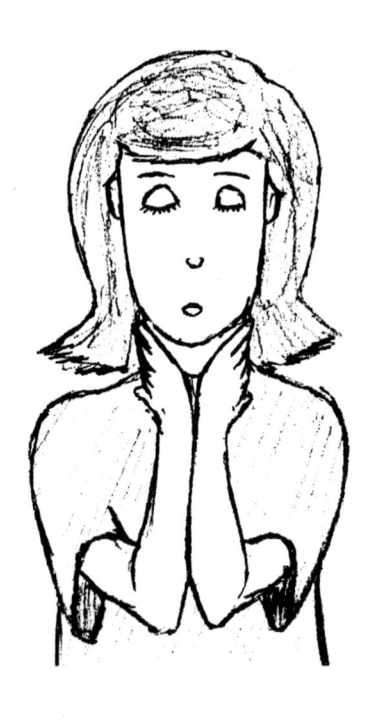

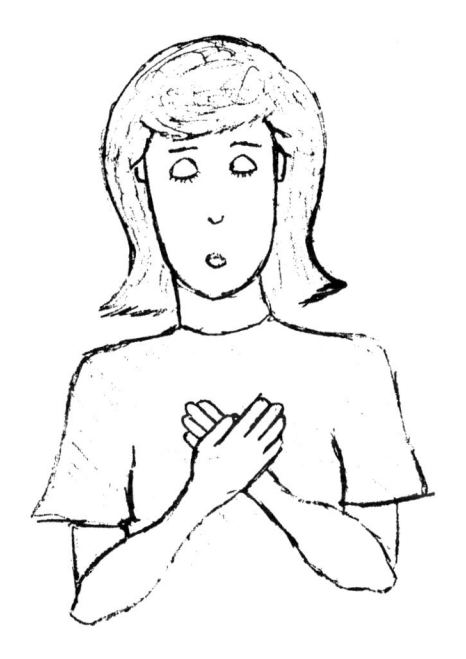

Allow a few moments at each position. Approximately two to three minutes per position is fine. Move your hands slowly and deliberately.

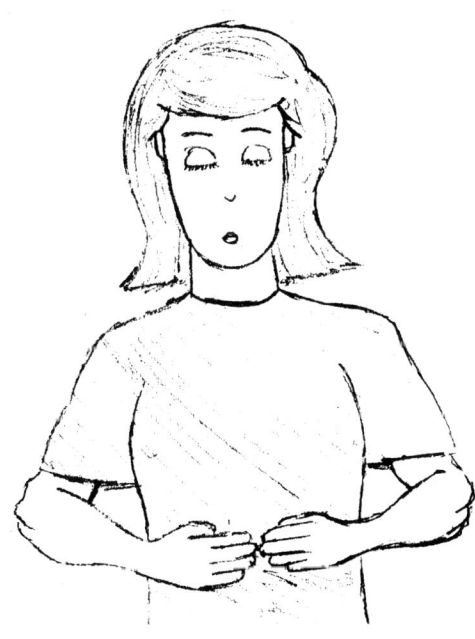

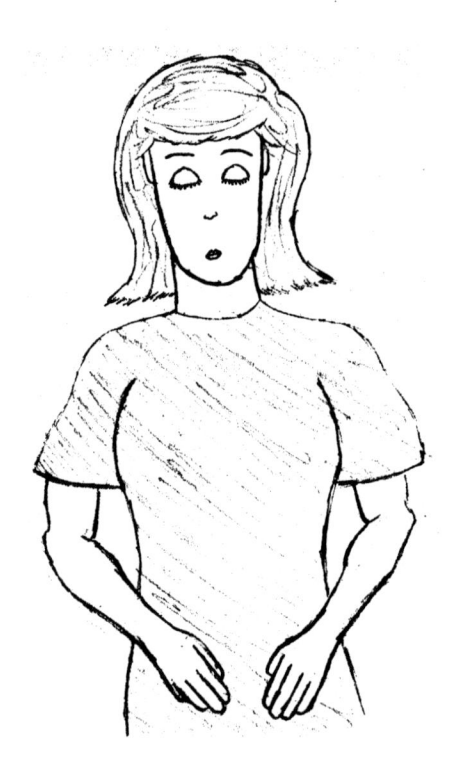

46   Healing: An Inner Awakening

Here your hands rest at the same level as your floating ribs. Then they move just above your hip bones.

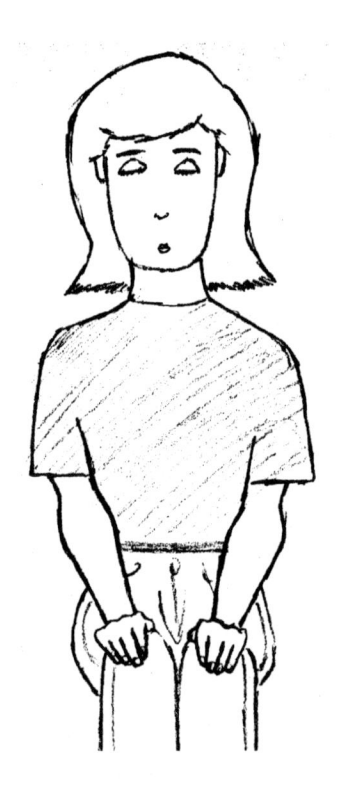

Allow both hands to rest on your knees. Then hold the ankles of each foot one at a time.

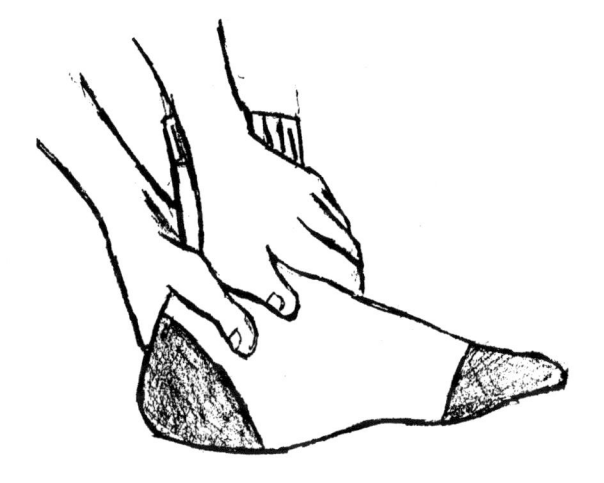

Then cradle both arches in your hands
of both feet, one foot at a time.

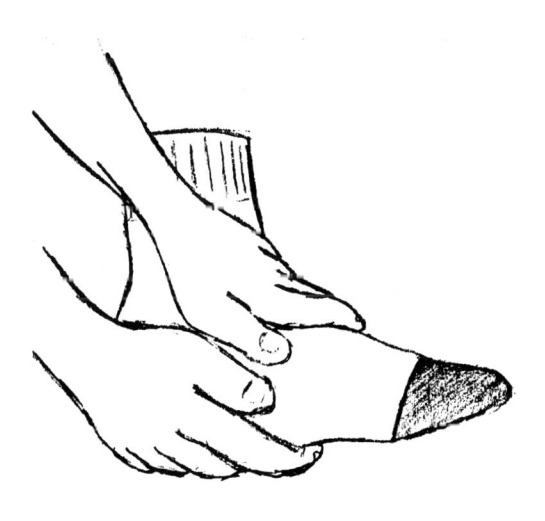

48   Healing: An Inner Awakening

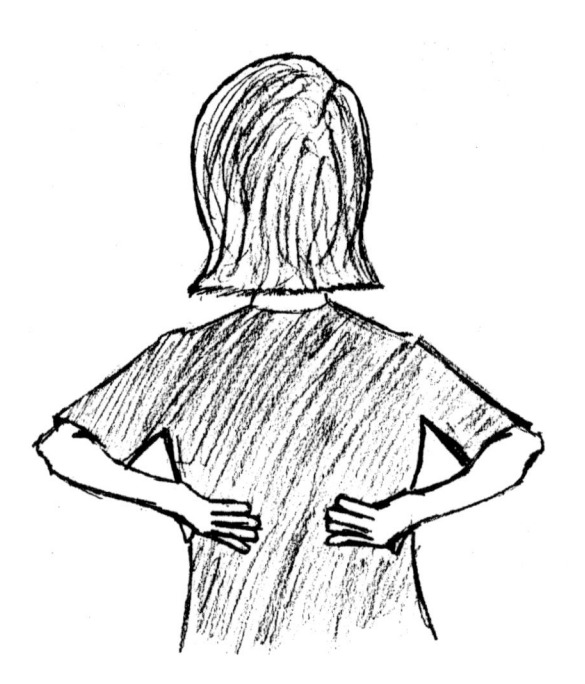

Completing this series of hand positions, allow yourself a short quite rest. Take a few moments for reflection and ease before jumping back into your day.

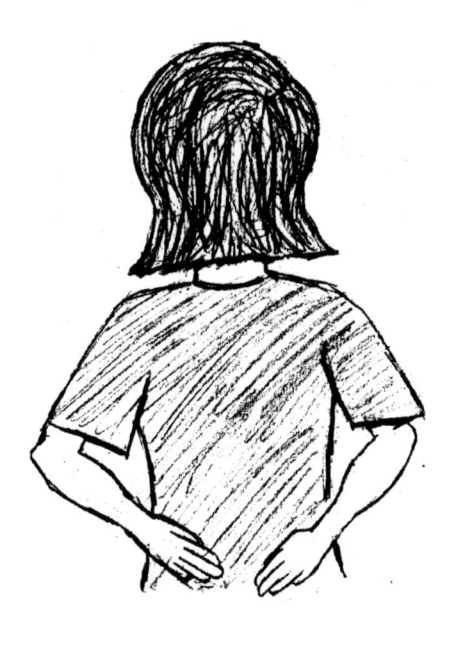

A session can last anywhere from 5 minutes to 2 hours, longer if facilitating during surgery. Upon completion release this person and bring yourself back to a conscious awareness of the room. As you release thank the person and allow the recipient to relax and absorb the experience. End the experience with a few moments of rest. When the person leaves, give yourself a moment to relax and re-hydrate[8].

I also recommend these sessions for horses, dogs, and other animals. I work with animal medical people too. We generate similar results to humans, and have raised a few eyebrows in amazement of a few veterinarian technicians and veterinarian doctors.

Basic Techniques

Directing

Directing is a technique for healing over distances. This distance can be as little as one inch or several miles. This is most appropriate during surgery, across a room, or walking through a shopping center.

Some believe this technique is best when pointing open palms towards the recipient.

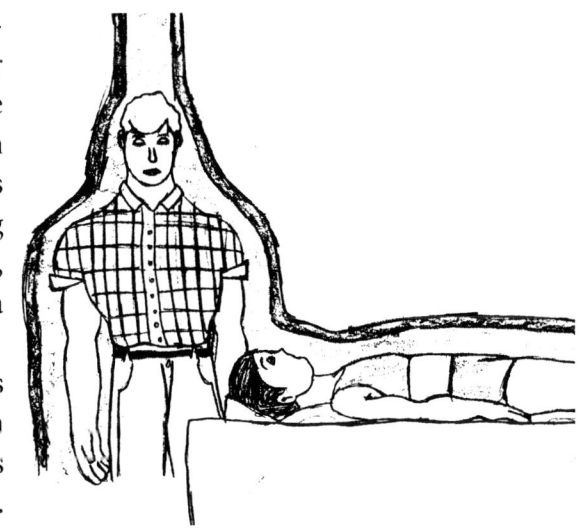

---

[8] Water is fine. Bio-magnetic healing is a work out too. For best results, drink something with electrolytes without sugar. Health food stores carry such waters, drinks, and supplement. Always check with your primary health care provider insuring in take of electrolytic drinks are safe for you before testing this suggestion.

Well if you are facilitating in a health care facility, it may create an uncomfortable situation, and if you are observing a 5-hour surgery, your arms are sure to tire. Since the catalyst is intention, any bio-magnetic healing propagates from the facilitator as a whole. Through sheer intention as little or large an area is affected.[9]

Standing or sitting normally in a relaxed position, or while walking, talking, or driving, the facilitator is a literal transponder for healing. As mentioned in the explanation, bio-magnetic healing is a form of electro-magnetic energy and the facilitator the conduit for this healing energy. Stand naturally, being present, and observe. This is what is necessary.

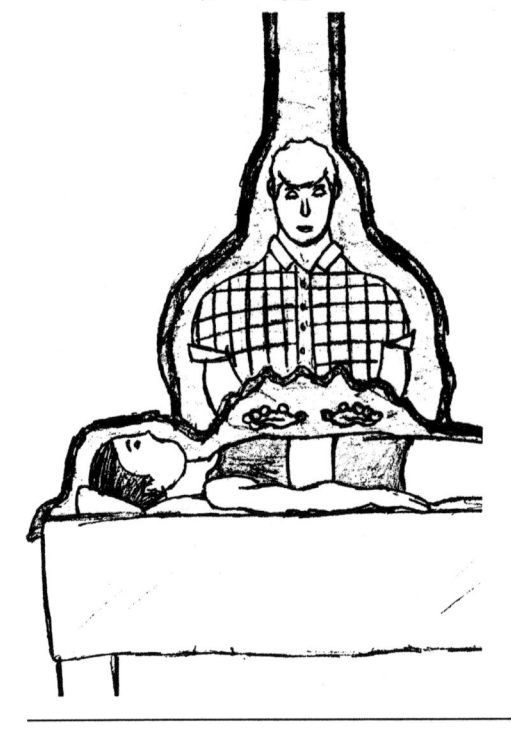

Sensing

A vital tool for the bio-magnetic healer is scanning. Hands open palms facing down beginning at the top of the head. Intently place all attention and focus in the palms of your hands. Slowly move your hands, being aware of any sensation(s), feelings, and even thoughts entering your mind. Slowly move your hands along the whole length of your friend, from head to feet. Repeat this movement from different levels away from the body; there is no

---

[9] During any course of facilitating the only intention should be that of healing. Healing what is for the best of the individual and all who is concerned. Remember healing is not about satisfying an egocentric goal. The only goal is the best experience for the individual requesting your facilitation.

physical contact with sensing. This assists in the discovery of areas requiring more attention.

A person need not be present for scanning. This works on a similar principle of Directing. However, it is receiving rather then facilitating. It is being aware of what is subtly present from the recipient. Scanning with this technique is best during medical procedures, especially surgery. At the printing of this book, we are welcome observers providing a service without physical contact during surgery. An actual full physical scan with your hands hovering about a doctor's patient can create a very interesting situation accompanied by some animated dialogue.

Group Healing

This technique creates a sense of communal purpose amongst practitioners. This is a good example of, "two heads are better than one." A group of licensed facilitators come together for a common interest, promoting healing—balance. It is the equivalent of a medical symposium, or ethical debate. Groups of similar professionals come together with intentions of promoting the highest good within their specialty. Meetings also include time for healing others. The person can be absent from the group.

Absentee Healing

Absentee healing is similar to group healing combined with beaming. It may take place alone or with a group of other facilitators. Physical or mental aids are incorporated increasing the facilitator's focus and awareness.

Vibration and Tapping

This method assists in balancing closed or excessive areas of energetic stimulation. They are similar to techniques utilized in Taoist healing methods. In an area requiring vibration, a facilitator's hand or finger oscillates. With Tapping, a fist or just a finger may tap a specific area. These techniques usually do not involve pounding or deep strikes as with the *Percussion* technique associated with Swedish massage. Again, this technique requires personal training with a licensed instructor.

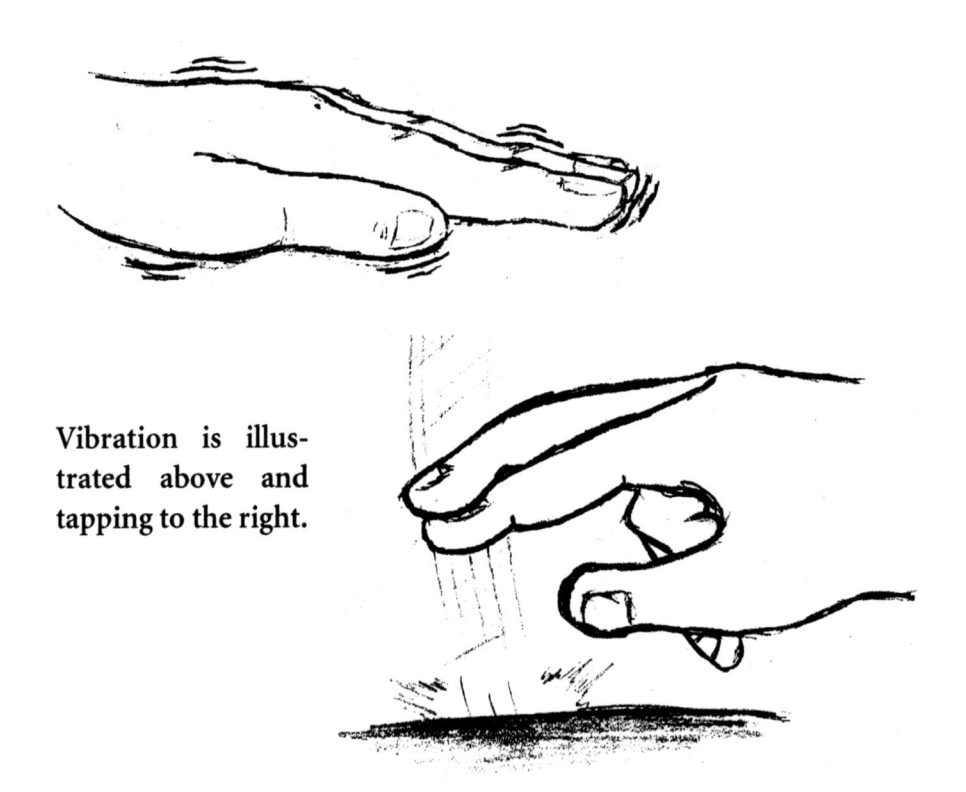

Vibration is illustrated above and tapping to the right.

Intention/Visualization, Verbalization and Action

Most esoteric schools stress the importance of thoughts, what one sees (eyes), and the breath or speech, and physical movements or actions as very powerful tools. Esoteric healers incorporate these tools ensuring the best for the individual requesting the session.

1) **Focusing**

This process focuses the practitioner's thoughts and intention for the matter at hand—balance. Here the practitioner prepares their mind for one of the most intimate contacts anyone can have with another human being–the purpose of restoring balance–healing.

A few surgeons I met usually practice a form of this before touching a scalpel. One medical doctor I work with reviews the surgical procedure in her mind before she scrubs up for surgery. Another surgeon I facilitated for actually touched the patient on the area to be operated, before it was sterilized of course, and became quite. I asked him what he was doing and he said quietly, "Praying."

2) Verbalizing

A word, speech, or a tone *reminds* the practitioner of their specific intention or goal for the session. In some instances, just the breath of the practitioner is considered empowered for it is fortified through their intention.

Even though the surgical team is aware of the procedure being done, the doctor usually discusses the procedure with those assisting, sometimes briefly, other times at length. This assures the patient is receiving the exact procedure necessary. The medical director of Convergences Institute always discusses with me the procedures she will execute, though I never physically touch the patient while in the surgery room.

3) Action

This is the actual physical movement or use of the body. This is the final ingredient for creating the physical reality of the original intention. In esoteric practices, it appears as an odd assortment of hand gestures. In everyday life it varies from taking a shower, doing laundry, physical exercise, injecting a life saving drug, to the physical placement of hands on another creating a greater sense of ease and caring.

This simple practice utilizing the tools built into our very makeup supported by authentic compassion, love, and tolerance (boddhicitta[10]) for others creates a sense of peace and balance beyond that of the customary practice of worry and complaining, or could it? Try it yourself. What small thing do you want from your day today? Think about what you want, and what you need to say to your self or others to generate this. It could be as simple as smiling and saying thank you to the next person you meet. Try it; you might just get what you want from your life.

---

[10] (Sanskrit) Awakened mind.

Afterword

Healing, what is it? People use this term freely without any heart full considerations. This very important process or state of being human is overlooked just as easily as the breath you just released. Whether you choose investigating esoteric healing as a profession or an integrative complement, take a few moments to review your inner motives and expectations. Spend a few moments with each question. Some are a bit ambiguous; fill in the details as they relate to your experience. This is only another first step.

- What is a Healer?
- What is Healing?
- Why do you wish to Heal?
- How do you wish to Heal?

About the Author

At a very early age, my parents provoked a fun filled exploration of self and the world. Raised in a typical religious tradition on the New Jersey side of the New York City Metropolitan area curiosity drew me towards Eastern cultures, martial arts, and spirituality. I began exploring meditation during late grammar school. At eighteen years of age, I officially began studying Japanese martial arts and esoteric meditation. My desire for understanding became insatiable leading me to a degree in Physics in one hand, a massage therapy certificate in the other, and on the road to Dayton, Ohio, were my martial and spiritual pursuits continued.

I encountered Reiki in the late 80's taking the first degree in April of 1991. Years latter, I received a Reiki teaching license, obtained certification as a holistic practitioner, stress management coach, and certified teacher of Japanese martial arts and esoteric mind science—the same mind sciences as the founder of Reiki has studied. The current medical director of Convergences Institute, Glenda Dahlquist MD, requested I facilitate Bio-magnetic healing, Reiki, for her patience. Almost five years later, after countless surgeries and medical procedures, Convergences Institute opens.

I hope in assisting as many people as possible with the few words placed in this book. I look forward to meeting and assisting those who attend our workshops and talks. Thank you for you interest and may your life be filled with clarity, peace, and ease.

Please feel free to contact me with any questions:
    Website: http://Welcome.to/Convergences.Institute
    E-mail: Convergences@usa.net

Mail: Convergences Institute
6 West Franklin Street
Bellbrook, OH 45305
USA
Phone: (937) 848-9875

Appendix A

Reiki: An Interpretation

Some circles of Reiki use the Japanese phonetic spelling for Reiki, many people continue using the Japanese kanji to the left of this paragraph. This Japanese set of characters actually contains four separate words. From top to bottom the characters read: rain, standing, or standing rain, and pressure and inside pressure is rice or rice under pressure. A modern Japanese person will interpret this top character, Rei, as spirit or ghost, and the bottom character, ki, as life energy, life essence, or spiritual energy. Therefore, we have ghost or spirit and life force or essence of life.

Modern Reiki facilitators define the characters Reiki as "Universal Life Force" though I feel this deserves more insight, or at least my modern western ego does. The bottom two characters rice under pressure, or life essence, or ki, evolved from ancient Japanese, stemming from an original Chinese character. If you have rice under pressure, or cooked rice, you ate, which assists in maintaining a healthy life. This is very clear, though the top character is a bit more obscure, in the presented context.

The top character, rei, is composed of standing or still, on the bottom and rain on top. I discovered the meaning came to be spirit or ghost due to the natural effect of standing rain. If you look at a heavy down pour of rain, it plays tricks with your eyes. It can appear something is present when it is not. Hence, the definition being spirit or ghost. With a bit more research and insight I though, spirit, heavy or spirited rain fall, this could be interpreted as a strong will or spirit. Though the actual definition is not, maybe the founder is being poetic as many old Japanese were in the martial arts labeling techniques. Martial artists would do this to capture the esoteric, or inner trick of performing the technique perfectly. Sometimes it is to hide a family secret so as preserving the life of the family. It is difficult to validate this hypothesis thought it makes greater personal sense. Having a great amount of spirit or being spirited, maybe Reiki is a motto of sorts too.

Rei, spirit or spirited, and ki life force or essence of manifesting life. A definition I enjoy is: If we approach life with a great spirit and determination. If we follow our heart's dream with great conviction and a proper motivation, and back this with the energy or the force that gives life, some say inner will, others call it ki or prana, and some call it the grace of God, we can accomplish that which we truly need, and the world is asking from us.

Appendix B

Sample intake form.

Name: _____ Phone( ) _____

Address: _____ Age: _____ Gender: M F

City: _____ State: _____

Referred by: _____ Referral's Telephone( ) _____

Emergence contact name: _____

Phone( ) _____ Circle all appropriate answers below:

Have you ever experienced a bio-magnetic healing session before: Yes No

If so how long ago: _____ How often do you receive sessions: _____

What is your goal for today's session: _____

_____

_____

Are you wearing contact lenses? Yes No

Are you currently under any holistic or medical care? Yes No

If Yes please briefly describe and list practitioner(s)' names and phone number:

_____

_____

_____

Please list any questions or concerns you have:

_____

_____

Intentional Healing™ or any form of bio-magnetic healing has not been proven contraindicated for any medical condition or specific condition, but a referral from your primary care physician may be required before service being provided. I am also aware that touch maybe required during this session. I consent to any touch, though if I feel uncomfortable at any point during the session I can and will terminate the session. All information is held in strict confidentiality.

Client Signature _____ Date: _____

Practitioner Signature _____ Date: _____

> **Consent to Treatment of Minor:** By my signature below, I hereby authorize _____
>
> to administer bio-magnetic/Reiki, or somatic therapy techniques to my child or dependent as they deem necessary.
>
> Signature of Parent or Guardian_____ Date: _____

© Copyright Convergences Institute 1998, 1999, 2000

©Copyright David A. Piser 1998, 1999, 2000

Appendix C

Healing Protocol

1. Center
2. Intent
3. Create Space
4. Permission
5. Protect
6. Envision
7. Connect
8. Facilitate
9. Offer
10. Thank
11. Disconnect
12. Release
13. Thank
14. Center
15. Reflect

*   *   *

Appendix D

Our Programs at Convergences Institute

Each programs moves the individual towards greater competency as a facilitator. Your knowledge and experience grow within the topics of bio-magnetic healing and personal holistic methods. We look forward to seeing you at our center or a locally sponsored workshop! Thank you.

Intentional Healing™ Curriculum

      I). Certified Intentional Healing Practitioner
      II). Certified Intentional Healing Practitioner II
      III). Certified Intentional Healing Senior Practitioner
      IV). Certified Intentional Healing Senior Practitioner II
      V). Certified Intentional Healing Instructor

Reiki Licensing Program

Level 1 Licensed Practitioner
Rki 100 Reiki Level 1
Med 100 Meditation (Centering)
Med 200 Meditation (Insight)
Rki 101 Clinical Practical

Level 2 Licensed Practitioner
Rki 200 Reiki Level 2
Rki 220 Eastern and Western Anatomy & Physiology
Les 100 Personal Awareness Matrix
(Apt230 Allopathic Protocol) only for medical electives
Rki 201 Clinical Practical

Licensed Senior Practitioner
Rki 300 Reiki Level 3
Med 300 Advanced Meditation (Following)
Rki 301 Clinical Practical
Approved Elective

Licensed Master Practitioner
Rki 400 Reiki Level 4
LES 200 Personal Awareness Matrix II

Rki 401 Clinical Practical
Approved Elective

Licensed Teacher
Rki 500 Reiki Level 5
Rki 501 Clinical Practical
Rki 501 Assisting internship
Rki 501 Primary internship
Rki 600 Independent Study

Notes:

Notes:

Notes:

Notes:

Notes:

Notes:

Notes:

Notes:

Notes:

Notes:

Notes:

Notes:

Notes:

9 780595 141548